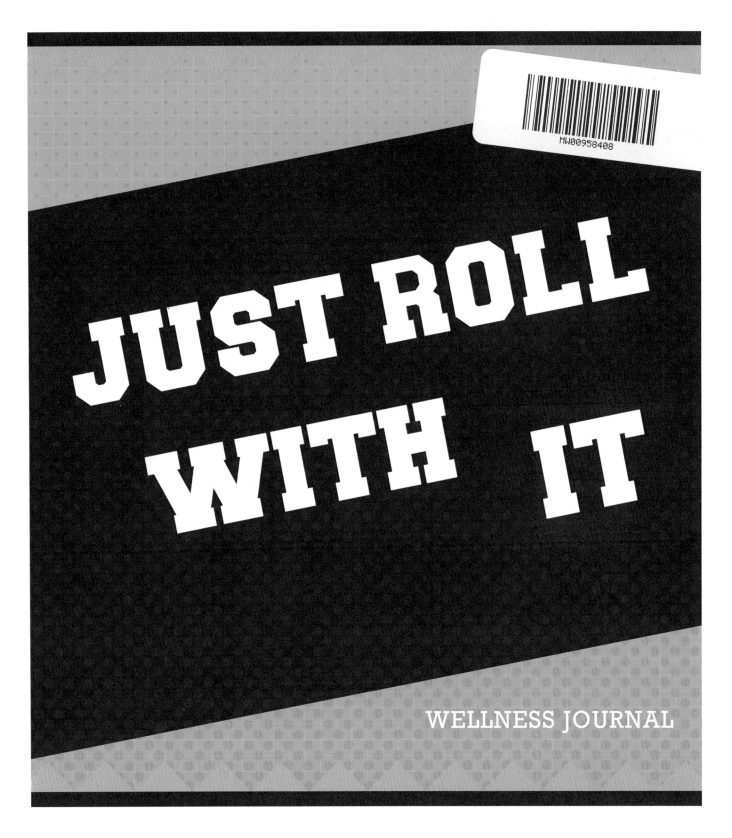

JUST ROLL WITH IT

WELLNESS JOURNAL

We can't stop the waves, but we can learn how to surf. -Jon Kabat-Zinn

Sarah Plummer Taylor, MSW, & Kate Hendricks Thomas, PhD

Just Roll With It Wellness 30-day Lifestyle Journal
By Sarah Plummer Taylor and Kate Hendricks Thomas

Published by Resilience Press, A Division of Just Roll With It Wellness LLC, Tuscaloosa AL.

Plummer Taylor, Sarah
Hendricks Thomas, Kate

ISBN13: 9781502594761
ISBN10: 1502594765

Front and back cover design: Make My Notebook, Sara Blette, www.MakeMyNotebook.com

Printed in the United States of America

10 9 8 7 6 5 4 3 2 1

INTRODUCTION

At Just Roll With It Wellness, we are dedicated to helping you build a strong body, a focused mind, an open spirit, and a practice of gratitude.
We want you to craft a sustainably healthy life that you actually enjoy!

Consider this a place to capture the details of your journey as a wellness warrior. Let this journal empower you to create sustainable lifestyle changes. Write down your goals, track your progress, and feel those changes bring vitality to your life!

This journal is your guide to vibrant living and fulfilling nourishment so you can achieve a state of optimal wellbeing despite the daily stresses and setbacks that might normally get in your way.

Self-care builds resilience! Do this for you, as well as recognize how your improved self-care impacts your relationship with others.

How you think, how you breathe, how you move, how you work, and how you love all impacts your health, too. In truth, food is not the only thing that feeds us.

You want your life to be gratefully full, don't you? You want to feel satisfied, joyful, and like you're making a difference in this world, right? Well, we want to help you live that happy, healthy, and successful life of purpose; utilizing this journal is one big step in that direction!

The cool thing is that our body, mind, and spirit have the ability to work together to help us bring the best version of our self to every day, every relationship, and every challenge.

Our body has an innate intelligence to keep itself healthy. Unfortunately, many of us are bombarded and confused by pervasive stress, trauma, or unhealthy environments. Given half a chance, the body will heal the body; the body will serve the body; the body will empower the body to thrive. But we must give it that chance.

Beyond the body, we need to keep the mind and spirit healthy, too, though, don't we?

Cultivating awareness allows us to tap into that innate mental and spiritual intelligence, too. Awareness can be cultivated through journaling, practicing, and applying healthy principles. Psalm 46:10 really applies here – we have to get quiet to hear our biggest callings and dreams. "Be still and know …"

This journal is designed to educate, empower, guide and encourage you on your quest to better health in body, mind, and spirit.

Enjoy the journey, dream big, take action, and ultimately, Just Roll With It!

"HEALING DOESN'T MEAN ACHIEVING PERFECTION OR 'FIXING' YOURSELF. HEALING IS A PROCESS AND A PRACTICE."

-SARAH PLUMMER TAYLOR, MSW
Just Roll With It: 7 Battle Tested Truths for Building a Resilient Life

HOW TO USE THIS JOURNAL

"A journey of a thousand miles begins with a single step." —Lao Tzu

Before you dive right into this goodness, you probably want to know what the Just Roll With It method is all about, right? Simply put, *Just Roll With It* means learning to surf when the waves keep coming, going with the flow, living from your truly-aligned core character traits and being flexible, being grateful even in the eye of the storm, and building the resiliency that will allow you to live the life you love and love the life you live.

DO THIS

HAVE FAITH – It'll all be ok. Take heart, let go and let God, go with the flow and trust that your body does know how to fulfill its natural purpose and reach optimal health. The more you invest in your own journey, the more reward you will reap.

BE SINCERE – Being authentic is key. This stack of paper won't do a darn bit of good if you're not authentic, raw, and vulnerable. It's your journal, so use it how you want to! Keep it private and use it like a personal diary, or simply use it as a log of information to guide your adjustments and successes moving forward.

BE ENGAGED & EXCITED – In other words, be present and be dynamic! Do your best to be fully engaged while making notes or journaling because the more "here" you are, the more you'll get out of it. Also, don't feel like you've got to do this all on your own. "Every success story includes others. Don't be afraid to ask for help," from *Just Roll With It: 7 Battle Tested Truths for Building a Resilient Life*. See, your authors are a couple of smarty-pants who are also fun-loving and we've developed this journal with you in mind! But heck, if you want to spice it up or skip some spots, go for it. Don't feel like you've got to roll inside the lines at all times.

BE PERSISTENT - If you miss a day, no worries. Pick up where you left off whenever you can. Stick with it, and we promise you'll be glad you did when you see how much awesome stuff has happened since you started the journal.

WITH THESE

THE WISH LIST – Your wishes, your dreams, your desires are the "why" behind the effort you're making and why you've bothered to open this journal each day. You're not putting your wishes in the "nice-to-have" box anymore. Write them down and be stoked when you see them start to blossom.

AM PAGE – A space for your morning intentions. Set aside time at the beginning of the day to process and absorb your initial feelings, make a short gratitude list, then set your goals. This could take 5 minutes or 30 depending on your preference. Determine what best serves you. Carving out this time first thing helps you set a solid foundation for the rest of your day.

PM PAGE – A space for your evening reflections. Utilize quiet time to be present, consider how your day went, note what felt like "wins," observe what felt like "losses," and record what you are grateful for that happened that day. Honoring this time, and writing each night, conditions your mind and body to slow down and prepare for sleep, often resulting in better rest.

WEEKLY CHECK-INS & GUIDED EXERCISES – These exercises open up different parts of your mind and spirit to motivate you to deepen your journey beyond the tangible. We're aiming for small, sustainable changes, right? But sometimes those are hard to notice, so these check-ins are great places to take stock and give yourself a well-deserved pat on the back.

TERMS –The daily pages include space to check healthy habits you've accomplished. Feel free to add your own categories of healthy to-do's, too. The following page provides explanations of terms we included.

"WE ARE WIRED TO CONNECT WITH GOD AND WITH EACH OTHER."

DR. KATE HENDRICKS THOMAS,
Brave, Strong, And True: The Modern Warrior's Battle For Balance

TERMS

SET THE MOOD = Morning intentions – did you fill in the AM Journal page?

COOK LIKE A GROWN UP = Home-cooked food ___x meals – cooking your own food at home is better for your wallet and your waistline! Did you eat out or cook for yourself today?

EAT LIKE A GROWN UP = Mindful eating – slowing down while eating is one of the simplest gifts we can give ourselves to aid with digestion and reduce stress. Studies show that we absorb nutrients differently when we eat mindfully. That salad in front of a television doesn't deliver the same amount of iron as the exact same salad consumed mindfully at the table. Did you scarf? Did you watch television or look at your phone while eating? That doesn't count as mindful, my friend.

EAT A LITTLE LESS OF _____ = Reduced one food – did you consume one less serving perhaps of sugar, processed food, junk food, meat, caffeine, or something you're trying to minimize? You don't have to move in leaps and bounds here! Remember, small sustainable changes make the biggest impact.

PRACTICE SELF-CARE = Did you do something for yourself that increased your health and happiness?

BREATHE MINDFULLY = Conscious breathing – carving out little moments throughout the day to inhale and exhale deeply, smoothly, and mindfully. This can do a world of wonder for your stress levels. Plus, neuroscience is showing that 3-15 minutes of mindful breathwork each day can rewire your gray matter and improve your working memory capacity. Want to be smarter and more emotionally-regulated? Try it!

ENJOY THE GREAT OUTDOORS = Fresh air – Please, tell us you haven't been inside all day. We are creatures designed to move and breathe outside. Did you get some today (fresh air, that is)?

MOVE MORE = Physical activity – Movement is medicine. Did you take your prescription today? It may feel hard to get out the door, but you'll feel better once you do!

CONNECT SPIRITUALLY = Prayer/meditation – Maybe this overlaps with your morning intentions or breath work? Either way, did you take some time to sit and think consciously and co-create with your Divine?

CONNECT SOCIALLY = We are social creatures by nature, whether introverted, extroverted, or a mix of both personality types. Your definition of "meaningful connection" may be different than ours, but did you take time in some capacity to reach out today? Studies show that social support adds an average of 7.5 years to your life; let a little love in for your health!

EMBRACE MY OFFICE SPACE = Whether you work from home or outside of it, that space impacts your health. Your office space includes the work you do, the people with whom you interact, and your physical environment itself. Did you enjoy your office space today?

RECEIVE TOUCH = Touch/massage/body work – Behold, the power of touch! Because we are little animals at heart, we like to be petted, too. Touch and massage can go a long way toward relieving stress and helping your body and brain function smoothly.

EXPERIENCE HAPPINESS = Get yourself some joy! – Laughter can be "the best medicine," or "the simplest meditation." How much happiness did you get in your world today?

HONOR ME TIME = Time to yourself – as social as we are, we need alone time to recharge and realign. Did you get your "me time" today?

VISUALIZE MY FUTURE = The power of visualization is for real! Professional athletes use it, top executives use it, and regular folks use it, too. Set your goals and map out your path to health and success.

GET A GOOD NIGHT'S SLEEP = Seriously SLEEP! Quality over quantity. Turn off stimulating electronics an hour before bed, avoid caffeine after 2pm, and remember to create a cozy sleep space - beds are for sex or sleeping, nothing else.

THE CIRCLE OF LIFE

What does YOUR life look like?

1. Place a dot in each category slice to indicate your level of satisfaction within each area. Place a dot at the center of the circle to indicate dissatisfaction, or on the periphery to indicate satisfaction. Most people fall somewhere in between (see example).

2. Connect the dots to see your Circle of Life.

3. Identify imbalances. Determine where to spend more time and energy to create balance.

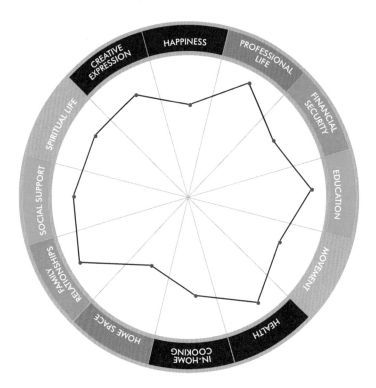

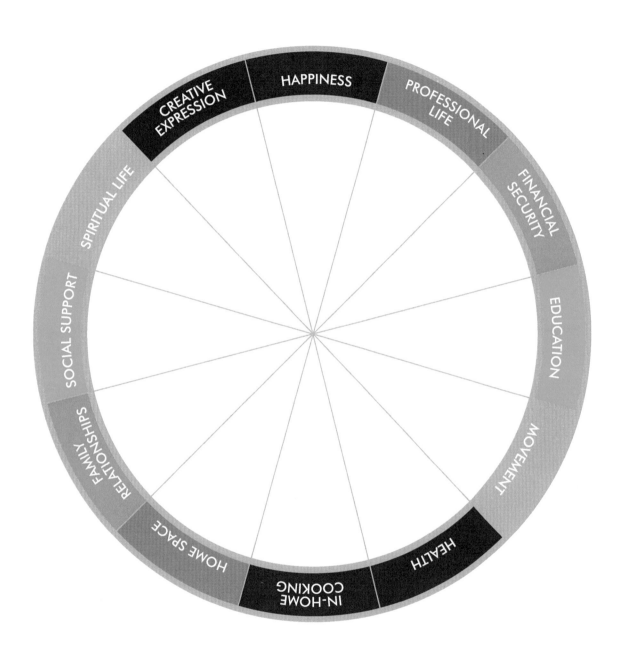

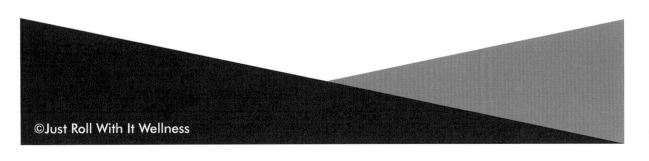

DREAM LIST

This is your space to dream.

Make a list of what you wish would happen in the next 30 days. Dream big and work your way toward smaller, more definable goals. When they happen, check the box off to the right, and write a small reflection of gratitude for having realized your dream.

> "You are never too old to set another goal or to dream a new dream."
> - C.S. Lewis

	DREAM	DONE	REFLECTION
1			
2			
3			
4			
5			
6			
7			
8			
9			
10			
11			

"JOURNALING OR EXPRESSIVE WRITING IS A SIMPLE, GENTLE, AND INEXPENSIVE HEALING TECHNIQUE. I CONSIDER IT A POWERFUL THERAPEUTIC TOOL TO LEARN MORE ABOUT YOURSELF AND BECOME AWARE OF HOW YOUR MIND AND EMOTIONS CAN INFLUENCE YOU PHYSICALLY."

-DR ANDREW WEIL

AM JOURNAL

Rolled out of bed. Today my outlook, mood, and/or intentions are:

3 Goals to roll with today and the steps to get there:

| 1. | 2. | 3. |

| A.

B.

C. | A.

B.

C. | A.

B.

C. |

Plans for fun, chill-time, or adventures today:

3 Things I am grateful for:

PM JOURNAL

Today I made time to:

o Set the mood
o Cook like a grown up
o Eat like a grown up
o Eat a little less of…
o Practice self-care
o Breathe mindfully

o Enjoy the great outdoors
o Move more
o Connect spiritually
o Connect socially
o Embrace my office space

o Recieve touch
o Experience Happiness
o Honor "me time"
o Visualize my future
o Get a good night's sleep

How much of the good stuff did I get today?

Water/hydration _____
Whole Grains _____
Veggies _____
Fruit _____

Healthy Fat _____
Protein _____
Supplements _____

How did I roll today? Thumbs up, down, or somewhere in between?

Mood _____
Energy _____

Digestion _____
Cravings _____

Today, I appreciate myself because:

Today, I added-in or crowded-out:

Choices that did not really serve or support me:

Happy, grateful, or loving thoughts before bed-time:

AM JOURNAL

Rolled out of bed. Today my outlook, mood, and/or intentions are:

3 Goals to roll with today and the steps to get there:

1.	2.	3.

A. B. C.	A. B. C.	A. B. C.

Plans for fun, chill-time, or adventures today:

3 Things I am grateful for:

PM JOURNAL

Today I made time to:

- o Set the mood
- o Cook like a grown up
- o Eat like a grown up
- o Eat a little less of…
- o Practice self-care
- o Breathe mindfully

- o Enjoy the great outdoors
- o Move more
- o Connect spiritually
- o Connect socially
- o Embrace my office space

- o Recieve touch
- o Experience Happiness
- o Honor "me time"
- o Visualize my future
- o Get a good night's sleep

How much of the good stuff did I get today?

Water/hydration _____

Whole Grains _____

Veggies _____

Fruit _____

Healthy Fat _____

Protein _____

Supplements _____

How did I roll today? Thumbs up, down, or somewhere in between?

Mood _____

Energy _____

Digestion _____

Cravings _____

Today, I appreciate myself because:

Today, I added-in or crowded-out:

Choices that did not really serve or support me:

Happy, grateful, or loving thoughts before bed-time:

AM JOURNAL

Rolled out of bed. Today my outlook, mood, and/or intentions are:

3 Goals to roll with today and the steps to get there:

| 1. | 2. | 3. |

| A.

B.

C. | A.

B.

C. | A.

B.

C. |

Plans for fun, chill-time, or adventures today:

3 Things I am grateful for:

PM JOURNAL

Today I made time to:

o Set the mood

o Cook like a grown up

o Eat like a grown up

o Eat a little less of…

o Practice self-care

o Breathe mindfully

o Enjoy the great outdoors

o Move more

o Connect spiritually

o Connect socially

o Embrace my office space

o Recieve touch

o Experience Happiness

o Honor "me time"

o Visualize my future

o Get a good night's sleep

How much of the good stuff did I get today?

Water/hydration _____

Whole Grains _____

Veggies _____

Fruit _____

Healthy Fat _____

Protein _____

Supplements _____

How did I roll today? Thumbs up, down, or somewhere in between?

Mood _____

Energy _____

Digestion _____

Cravings _____

Today, I appreciate myself because:

Today, I added-in or crowded-out:

Choices that did not really serve or support me:

Happy, grateful, or loving thoughts before bed-time:

AM JOURNAL

Rolled out of bed. Today my outlook, mood, and/or intentions are:

3 Goals to roll with today and the steps to get there:

1.	2.	3.

A. B. C.	A. B. C.	A. B. C.

Plans for fun, chill-time, or adventures today:

3 Things I am grateful for:

PM JOURNAL

Today I made time to:

- o Set the mood
- o Cook like a grown up
- o Eat like a grown up
- o Eat a little less of…
- o Practice self-care
- o Breathe mindfully

- o Enjoy the great outdoors
- o Move more
- o Connect spiritually
- o Connect socially
- o Embrace my office space

- o Recieve touch
- o Experience Happiness
- o Honor "me time"
- o Visualize my future
- o Get a good night's sleep

How much of the good stuff did I get today?

Water/hydration ————————————

Whole Grains ————————————

Veggies ————————————

Fruit ————————————

Healthy Fat ————————————

Protein ————————————

Supplements ————————————

How did I roll today? Thumbs up, down, or somewhere in between?

Mood ————————————

Energy ————————————

Digestion ————————————

Cravings ————————————

Today, I appreciate myself because:

Today, I added-in or crowded-out:

Choices that did not really serve or support me:

Happy, grateful, or loving thoughts before bed-time:

AM JOURNAL

Rolled out of bed. Today my outlook, mood, and/or intentions are:

3 Goals to roll with today and the steps to get there:

1.	2.	3.

A. B. C.	A. B. C.	A. B. C.

Plans for fun, chill-time, or adventures today:

3 Things I am grateful for:

PM JOURNAL

Today I made time to:

o Set the mood

o Cook like a grown up

o Eat like a grown up

o Eat a little less of…

o Practice self-care

o Breathe mindfully

o Enjoy the great outdoors

o Move more

o Connect spiritually

o Connect socially

o Embrace my office space

o Recieve touch

o Experience Happiness

o Honor "me time"

o Visualize my future

o Get a good night's sleep

How much of the good stuff did I get today?

Water/hydration ─────────────

Whole Grains ─────────────

Veggies ─────────────

Fruit ─────────────

Healthy Fat ─────────────

Protein ─────────────

Supplements ─────────────

How did I roll today? Thumbs up, down, or somewhere in between?

Mood ─────────────

Energy ─────────────

Digestion ─────────────

Cravings ─────────────

Today, I appreciate myself because:

Today, I added-in or crowded-out:

Choices that did not really serve or support me:

Happy, grateful, or loving thoughts before bed-time:

DATE:

AM JOURNAL

Rolled out of bed. Today my outlook, mood, and/or intentions are:

Boxed area

3 Goals to roll with today and the steps to get there:

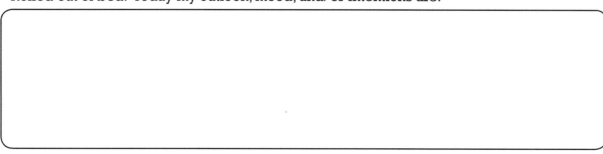

1.

2.

3.

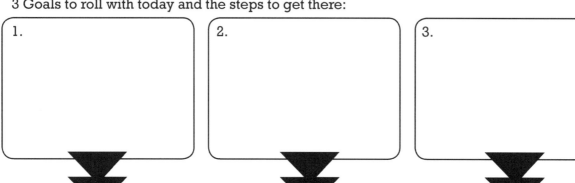

A.

B.

C.

A.

B.

C.

A.

B.

C.

Plans for fun, chill-time, or adventures today:

3 Things I am grateful for:

PM JOURNAL

Today I made time to:

- o Set the mood
- o Cook like a grown up
- o Eat like a grown up
- o Eat a little less of…
- o Practice self-care
- o Breathe mindfully

- o Enjoy the great outdoors
- o Move more
- o Connect spiritually
- o Connect socially
- o Embrace my office space

- o Recieve touch
- o Experience Happiness
- o Honor "me time"
- o Visualize my future
- o Get a good night's sleep

How much of the good stuff did I get today?

Water/hydration ————————	Healthy Fat ————————
Whole Grains ————————	Protein ————————
Veggies ————————	Supplements ————————
Fruit ————————	

How did I roll today? Thumbs up, down, or somewhere in between?

Mood ————————	Digestion ————————
Energy ————————	Cravings ————————

Today, I appreciate myself because:

Today, I added-in or crowded-out:

Choices that did not really serve or support me:

Happy, grateful, or loving thoughts before bed-time:

AM JOURNAL

Rolled out of bed. Today my outlook, mood, and/or intentions are:

3 Goals to roll with today and the steps to get there:

1.	2.	3.

A.	A.	A.
B.	B.	B.
C.	C.	C.

Plans for fun, chill-time, or adventures today:

3 Things I am grateful for:

PM JOURNAL

Today I made time to:

o Set the mood
o Cook like a grown up
o Eat like a grown up
o Eat a little less of…
o Practice self-care
o Breathe mindfully

o Enjoy the great outdoors
o Move more
o Connect spiritually
o Connect socially
o Embrace my office space

o Recieve touch
o Experience Happiness
o Honor "me time"
o Visualize my future
o Get a good night's sleep

How much of the good stuff did I get today?

Water/hydration _____
Whole Grains _____
Veggies _____
Fruit _____

Healthy Fat _____
Protein _____
Supplements _____

How did I roll today? Thumbs up, down, or somewhere in between?

Mood _____
Energy _____

Digestion _____
Cravings _____

Today, I appreciate myself because:

Today, I added-in or crowded-out:

Choices that did not really serve or support me:

Happy, grateful, or loving thoughts before bed-time:

WEEKLY AFTER ACTION REPORT

DATES _____

What's new? What's good?

Energy _____
_____

Digestion _____
_____

Cravings _____
_____

Hair & skin _____
_____

Mouth/teeth/tongue _____
_____

Body shape/body image/weight _____
_____

Breathing _____
_____

Moods _____
_____

Relationships _____

_____

Most nourishing food _____

_____

Most filling non-food _____

_____

Someone I especially appreciate _____

_____

Biggest challenge I faced _____

_____

Primary health concern _____

_____

Greatest success _____

_____

Most fun I had _____

_____

Something that became clear this week _____

_____

Other deep thoughts _____

_____

Next week is gonna roll like this…. _____

_____

AM JOURNAL

Rolled out of bed. Today my outlook, mood, and/or intentions are:

3 Goals to roll with today and the steps to get there:

1.	2.	3.

A.	A.	A.
B.	B.	B.
C.	C.	C.

Plans for fun, chill-time, or adventures today:

3 Things I am grateful for:

PM JOURNAL

Today I made time to:

o Set the mood
o Cook like a grown up
o Eat like a grown up
o Eat a little less of…
o Practice self-care
o Breathe mindfully

o Enjoy the great outdoors
o Move more
o Connect spiritually
o Connect socially
o Embrace my office space

o Recieve touch
o Experience Happiness
o Honor "me time"
o Visualize my future
o Get a good night's sleep

How much of the good stuff did I get today?

Water/hydration _____
Whole Grains _____
Veggies _____
Fruit _____

Healthy Fat _____
Protein _____
Supplements _____

How did I roll today? Thumbs up, down, or somewhere in between?

Mood _____
Energy _____

Digestion _____
Cravings _____

Today, I appreciate myself because:

Today, I added-in or crowded-out:

Choices that did not really serve or support me:

Happy, grateful, or loving thoughts before bed-time:

AM JOURNAL

Rolled out of bed. Today my outlook, mood, and/or intentions are:

3 Goals to roll with today and the steps to get there:

1.	2.	3.

A.	A.	A.
B.	B.	B.
C.	C.	C.

Plans for fun, chill-time, or adventures today:

3 Things I am grateful for:

PM JOURNAL

Today I made time to:

o Set the mood
o Cook like a grown up
o Eat like a grown up
o Eat a little less of...
o Practice self-care
o Breathe mindfully

o Enjoy the great outdoors
o Move more
o Connect spiritually
o Connect socially
o Embrace my office space

o Recieve touch
o Experience Happiness
o Honor "me time"
o Visualize my future
o Get a good night's sleep

How much of the good stuff did I get today?

Water/hydration _____
Whole Grains _____
Veggies _____
Fruit _____

Healthy Fat _____
Protein _____
Supplements _____

How did I roll today? Thumbs up, down, or somewhere in between?

Mood _____
Energy _____

Digestion _____
Cravings _____

Today, I appreciate myself because:

Today, I added-in or crowded-out:

Choices that did not really serve or support me:

Happy, grateful, or loving thoughts before bed-time:

AM JOURNAL

Rolled out of bed. Today my outlook, mood, and/or intentions are:

3 Goals to roll with today and the steps to get there:

1.	2.	3.

A.	A.	A.
B.	B.	B.
C.	C.	C.

Plans for fun, chill-time, or adventures today:

3 Things I am grateful for:

PM JOURNAL

Today I made time to:

o Set the mood
o Cook like a grown up
o Eat like a grown up
o Eat a little less of…
o Practice self-care
o Breathe mindfully

o Enjoy the great outdoors
o Move more
o Connect spiritually
o Connect socially
o Embrace my office space

o Recieve touch
o Experience Happiness
o Honor "me time"
o Visualize my future
o Get a good night's sleep

How much of the good stuff did I get today?

Water/hydration _____
Whole Grains _____
Veggies _____
Fruit _____

Healthy Fat _____
Protein _____
Supplements _____

How did I roll today? Thumbs up, down, or somewhere in between?

Mood _____
Energy _____

Digestion _____
Cravings _____

Today, I appreciate myself because:

Today, I added-in or crowded-out:

Choices that did not really serve or support me:

Happy, grateful, or loving thoughts before bed-time:

AM JOURNAL

Rolled out of bed. Today my outlook, mood, and/or intentions are:

3 Goals to roll with today and the steps to get there:

| 1. | 2. | 3. |

A.	A.	A.
B.	B.	B.
C.	C.	C.

Plans for fun, chill-time, or adventures today:

3 Things I am grateful for:

PM JOURNAL

Today I made time to:

- o Set the mood
- o Cook like a grown up
- o Eat like a grown up
- o Eat a little less of…
- o Practice self-care
- o Breathe mindfully

- o Enjoy the great outdoors
- o Move more
- o Connect spiritually
- o Connect socially
- o Embrace my office space

- o Recieve touch
- o Experience Happiness
- o Honor "me time"
- o Visualize my future
- o Get a good night's sleep

How much of the good stuff did I get today?

Water/hydration _____   Healthy Fat _____

Whole Grains _____   Protein _____

Veggies _____   Supplements _____

Fruit _____

How did I roll today? Thumbs up, down, or somewhere in between?

Mood _____   Digestion _____

Energy _____   Cravings _____

Today, I appreciate myself because:

Today, I added-in or crowded-out:

Choices that did not really serve or support me:

Happy, grateful, or loving thoughts before bed-time:

AM JOURNAL

Rolled out of bed. Today my outlook, mood, and/or intentions are:

3 Goals to roll with today and the steps to get there:

1.

2.

3.

A.

B.

C.

A.

B.

C.

A.

B.

C.

Plans for fun, chill-time, or adventures today:

3 Things I am grateful for:

PM JOURNAL

Today I made time to:

o Set the mood
o Cook like a grown up
o Eat like a grown up
o Eat a little less of...
o Practice self-care
o Breathe mindfully

o Enjoy the great outdoors
o Move more
o Connect spiritually
o Connect socially
o Embrace my office space

o Recieve touch
o Experience Happiness
o Honor "me time"
o Visualize my future
o Get a good night's sleep

How much of the good stuff did I get today?

Water/hydration _____

Whole Grains _____

Veggies _____

Fruit _____

Healthy Fat _____

Protein _____

Supplements _____

How did I roll today? Thumbs up, down, or somewhere in between?

Mood _____

Energy _____

Digestion _____

Cravings _____

Today, I appreciate myself because:

Today, I added-in or crowded-out:

Choices that did not really serve or support me:

Happy, grateful, or loving thoughts before bed-time:

AM JOURNAL

Rolled out of bed. Today my outlook, mood, and/or intentions are:

3 Goals to roll with today and the steps to get there:

| 1. | 2. | 3. |

A.	A.	A.
B.	B.	B.
C.	C.	C.

Plans for fun, chill-time, or adventures today:

3 Things I am grateful for:

PM JOURNAL

Today I made time to:

- o Set the mood
- o Cook like a grown up
- o Eat like a grown up
- o Eat a little less of…
- o Practice self-care
- o Breathe mindfully

- o Enjoy the great outdoors
- o Move more
- o Connect spiritually
- o Connect socially
- o Embrace my office space

- o Recieve touch
- o Experience Happiness
- o Honor "me time"
- o Visualize my future
- o Get a good night's sleep

How much of the good stuff did I get today?

Water/hydration	Healthy Fat	
Whole Grains	Protein	
Veggies	Supplements	
Fruit		

How did I roll today? Thumbs up, down, or somewhere in between?

Mood	Digestion	
Energy	Cravings	

Today, I appreciate myself because:

Today, I added-in or crowded-out:

Choices that did not really serve or support me:

Happy, grateful, or loving thoughts before bed-time:

AM JOURNAL

Rolled out of bed. Today my outlook, mood, and/or intentions are:

3 Goals to roll with today and the steps to get there:

1.	2.	3.

| A.

B.

C. | A.

B.

C. | A.

B.

C. |

Plans for fun, chill-time, or adventures today:

3 Things I am grateful for:

PM JOURNAL

Today I made time to:

- o Set the mood
- o Cook like a grown up
- o Eat like a grown up
- o Eat a little less of…
- o Practice self-care
- o Breathe mindfully

- o Enjoy the great outdoors
- o Move more
- o Connect spiritually
- o Connect socially
- o Embrace my office space

- o Recieve touch
- o Experience Happiness
- o Honor "me time"
- o Visualize my future
- o Get a good night's sleep

How much of the good stuff did I get today?

Water/hydration _____

Whole Grains _____

Veggies _____

Fruit _____

Healthy Fat _____

Protein _____

Supplements _____

How did I roll today? Thumbs up, down, or somewhere in between?

Mood _____

Energy _____

Digestion _____

Cravings _____

Today, I appreciate myself because:

Today, I added-in or crowded-out:

Choices that did not really serve or support me:

Happy, grateful, or loving thoughts before bed-time:

WEEKLY AFTER ACTION REPORT

DATES _____

What's new? What's good?

Energy _____

_____

Digestion _____

_____

Cravings _____

_____

Hair & skin _____

_____

Mouth/teeth/tongue _____

_____

Body shape/body image/weight _____

_____

Breathing _____

_____

Moods _____

_____

Relationships _____

_____

Most nourishing food _____

_____

Most filling non-food _____

_____

Someone I especially appreciate _____

_____

Biggest challenge I faced _____

_____

Primary health concern _____

_____

Greatest success _____

_____

Most fun I had _____

_____

Something that became clear this week _____

_____

Other deep thoughts _____

_____

Next week is gonna roll like this.... _____

_____

2 WEEK CHECK IN

It's been two weeks since you started this journey. Now is a good time to reflect on your progress and think about how you are moving toward your goals and dreams.

▶ Look back at the Dream List you created at the beginning of the journal. Which goal(s) are you closest to accomplishing?

▶ What got you there? Thinking about the Circle of Life, and daily practices this journal had guided you through, what has been helpful?

▶ What's left? What will help you reach your goal(s)?

▶ Which goals are you furthest from accomplishing?

▶ What may be holding you back?

▶ What are 1 or 2 things you can do right now to move you toward that goal?

dream on, dreamer...

AM JOURNAL

Rolled out of bed. Today my outlook, mood, and/or intentions are:

3 Goals to roll with today and the steps to get there:

1.	2.	3.

A. B. C.	A. B. C.	A. B. C.

Plans for fun, chill-time, or adventures today:

3 Things I am grateful for:

PM JOURNAL

Today I made time to:

o Set the mood
o Cook like a grown up
o Eat like a grown up
o Eat a little less of…
o Practice self-care
o Breathe mindfully

o Enjoy the great outdoors
o Move more
o Connect spiritually
o Connect socially
o Embrace my office space

o Recieve touch
o Experience Happiness
o Honor "me time"
o Visualize my future
o Get a good night's sleep

How much of the good stuff did I get today?

Water/hydration _____
Whole Grains _____
Veggies _____
Fruit _____

Healthy Fat _____
Protein _____
Supplements _____

How did I roll today? Thumbs up, down, or somewhere in between?

Mood _____
Energy _____

Digestion _____
Cravings _____

Today, I appreciate myself because:

Today, I added-in or crowded-out:

Choices that did not really serve or support me:

Happy, grateful, or loving thoughts before bed-time:

AM JOURNAL

Rolled out of bed. Today my outlook, mood, and/or intentions are:

3 Goals to roll with today and the steps to get there:

1.	2.	3.

A.	A.	A.
B.	B.	B.
C.	C.	C.

Plans for fun, chill-time, or adventures today:

3 Things I am grateful for:

PM JOURNAL

Today I made time to:

o Set the mood

o Cook like a grown up

o Eat like a grown up

o Eat a little less of…

o Practice self-care

o Breathe mindfully

o Enjoy the great outdoors

o Move more

o Connect spiritually

o Connect socially

o Embrace my office space

o Recieve touch

o Experience Happiness

o Honor "me time"

o Visualize my future

o Get a good night's sleep

How much of the good stuff did I get today?

Water/hydration _____

Whole Grains _____

Veggies _____

Fruit _____

Healthy Fat _____

Protein _____

Supplements _____

How did I roll today? Thumbs up, down, or somewhere in between?

Mood _____

Energy _____

Digestion _____

Cravings _____

Today, I appreciate myself because:

Today, I added-in or crowded-out:

Choices that did not really serve or support me:

Happy, grateful, or loving thoughts before bed-time:

AM JOURNAL

Rolled out of bed. Today my outlook, mood, and/or intentions are:

3 Goals to roll with today and the steps to get there:

| 1. | 2. | 3. |

| A.

B.

C. | A.

B.

C. | A.

B.

C. |

Plans for fun, chill-time, or adventures today:

3 Things I am grateful for:

PM JOURNAL

Today I made time to:

- o Set the mood
- o Cook like a grown up
- o Eat like a grown up
- o Eat a little less of…
- o Practice self-care
- o Breathe mindfully

- o Enjoy the great outdoors
- o Move more
- o Connect spiritually
- o Connect socially
- o Embrace my office space

- o Recieve touch
- o Experience Happiness
- o Honor "me time"
- o Visualize my future
- o Get a good night's sleep

How much of the good stuff did I get today?

Water/hydration _____   Healthy Fat _____

Whole Grains _____   Protein _____

Veggies _____   Supplements _____

Fruit _____

How did I roll today? Thumbs up, down, or somewhere in between?

Mood _____   Digestion _____

Energy _____   Cravings _____

Today, I appreciate myself because:

Today, I added-in or crowded-out:

Choices that did not really serve or support me:

Happy, grateful, or loving thoughts before bed-time:

AM JOURNAL

Rolled out of bed. Today my outlook, mood, and/or intentions are:

3 Goals to roll with today and the steps to get there:

1.	2.	3.

A.	A.	A.
B.	B.	B.
C.	C.	C.

Plans for fun, chill-time, or adventures today:

3 Things I am grateful for:

PM JOURNAL

Today I made time to:

o Set the mood
o Cook like a grown up
o Eat like a grown up
o Eat a little less of…
o Practice self-care
o Breathe mindfully

o Enjoy the great outdoors
o Move more
o Connect spiritually
o Connect socially
o Embrace my office space

o Recieve touch
o Experience Happiness
o Honor "me time"
o Visualize my future
o Get a good night's sleep

How much of the good stuff did I get today?

Water/hydration ⎯⎯⎯⎯⎯⎯⎯⎯⎯⎯⎯

Whole Grains ⎯⎯⎯⎯⎯⎯⎯⎯⎯⎯⎯

Veggies ⎯⎯⎯⎯⎯⎯⎯⎯⎯⎯⎯

Fruit ⎯⎯⎯⎯⎯⎯⎯⎯⎯⎯⎯

Healthy Fat ⎯⎯⎯⎯⎯⎯⎯⎯⎯⎯⎯

Protein ⎯⎯⎯⎯⎯⎯⎯⎯⎯⎯⎯

Supplements ⎯⎯⎯⎯⎯⎯⎯⎯⎯⎯⎯

How did I roll today? Thumbs up, down, or somewhere in between?

Mood ⎯⎯⎯⎯⎯⎯⎯⎯⎯⎯⎯

Energy ⎯⎯⎯⎯⎯⎯⎯⎯⎯⎯⎯

Digestion ⎯⎯⎯⎯⎯⎯⎯⎯⎯⎯⎯

Cravings ⎯⎯⎯⎯⎯⎯⎯⎯⎯⎯⎯

Today, I appreciate myself because:

Today, I added-in or crowded-out:

Choices that did not really serve or support me:

Happy, grateful, or loving thoughts before bed-time:

AM JOURNAL

Rolled out of bed. Today my outlook, mood, and/or intentions are:

3 Goals to roll with today and the steps to get there:

1.	2.	3.

A. B. C.	A. B. C.	A. B. C.

Plans for fun, chill-time, or adventures today:

3 Things I am grateful for:

PM JOURNAL

Today I made time to:

- o Set the mood
- o Cook like a grown up
- o Eat like a grown up
- o Eat a little less of...
- o Practice self-care
- o Breathe mindfully

- o Enjoy the great outdoors
- o Move more
- o Connect spiritually
- o Connect socially
- o Embrace my office space

- o Recieve touch
- o Experience Happiness
- o Honor "me time"
- o Visualize my future
- o Get a good night's sleep

How much of the good stuff did I get today?

Water/hydration ——————————

Whole Grains ——————————

Veggies ——————————

Fruit ——————————

Healthy Fat ——————————

Protein ——————————

Supplements ——————————

How did I roll today? Thumbs up, down, or somewhere in between?

Mood ——————————

Energy ——————————

Digestion ——————————

Cravings ——————————

Today, I appreciate myself because:

Today, I added-in or crowded-out:

Choices that did not really serve or support me:

Happy, grateful, or loving thoughts before bed-time:

AM JOURNAL

Rolled out of bed. Today my outlook, mood, and/or intentions are:

3 Goals to roll with today and the steps to get there:

| 1. | 2. | 3. |

| A.

B.

C. | A.

B.

C. | A.

B.

C. |

Plans for fun, chill-time, or adventures today:

3 Things I am grateful for:

PM JOURNAL

Today I made time to:

o Set the mood

o Cook like a grown up

o Eat like a grown up

o Eat a little less of...

o Practice self-care

o Breathe mindfully

o Enjoy the great outdoors

o Move more

o Connect spiritually

o Connect socially

o Embrace my office space

o Recieve touch

o Experience Happiness

o Honor "me time"

o Visualize my future

o Get a good night's sleep

How much of the good stuff did I get today?

Water/hydration ⎯⎯⎯⎯⎯⎯⎯⎯⎯⎯

Whole Grains ⎯⎯⎯⎯⎯⎯⎯⎯⎯⎯

Veggies ⎯⎯⎯⎯⎯⎯⎯⎯⎯⎯

Fruit ⎯⎯⎯⎯⎯⎯⎯⎯⎯⎯

Healthy Fat ⎯⎯⎯⎯⎯⎯⎯⎯⎯⎯

Protein ⎯⎯⎯⎯⎯⎯⎯⎯⎯⎯

Supplements ⎯⎯⎯⎯⎯⎯⎯⎯⎯⎯

How did I roll today? Thumbs up, down, or somewhere in between?

Mood ⎯⎯⎯⎯⎯⎯⎯⎯⎯⎯

Energy ⎯⎯⎯⎯⎯⎯⎯⎯⎯⎯

Digestion ⎯⎯⎯⎯⎯⎯⎯⎯⎯⎯

Cravings ⎯⎯⎯⎯⎯⎯⎯⎯⎯⎯

Today, I appreciate myself because:

Today, I added-in or crowded-out:

Choices that did not really serve or support me:

Happy, grateful, or loving thoughts before bed-time:

AM JOURNAL

Rolled out of bed. Today my outlook, mood, and/or intentions are:

3 Goals to roll with today and the steps to get there:

1.	2.	3.

A. B. C.	A. B. C.	A. B. C.

Plans for fun, chill-time, or adventures today:

3 Things I am grateful for:

PM JOURNAL

Today I made time to:

- o Set the mood
- o Cook like a grown up
- o Eat like a grown up
- o Eat a little less of...
- o Practice self-care
- o Breathe mindfully

- o Enjoy the great outdoors
- o Move more
- o Connect spiritually
- o Connect socially
- o Embrace my office space

- o Recieve touch
- o Experience Happiness
- o Honor "me time"
- o Visualize my future
- o Get a good night's sleep

How much of the good stuff did I get today?

Water/hydration _____

Whole Grains _____

Veggies _____

Fruit _____

Healthy Fat _____

Protein _____

Supplements _____

How did I roll today? Thumbs up, down, or somewhere in between?

Mood _____

Energy _____

Digestion _____

Cravings _____

Today, I appreciate myself because:

Today, I added-in or crowded-out:

Choices that did not really serve or support me:

Happy, grateful, or loving thoughts before bed-time:

WEEKLY AFTER ACTION REPORT

DATES _____

What's new? What's good?

Energy _____
_____

Digestion _____
_____

Cravings _____
_____

Hair & skin _____
_____

Mouth/teeth/tongue _____
_____

Body shape/body image/weight _____
_____

Breathing _____
_____

Moods _____
_____

Relationships _____

_____

Most nourishing food _____

_____

Most filling non-food _____

_____

Someone I especially appreciate _____

_____

Biggest challenge I faced _____

_____

Primary health concern _____

_____

Greatest success _____

_____

Most fun I had _____

_____

Something that became clear this week _____

_____

Other deep thoughts _____

_____

Next week is gonna roll like this.... _____

_____

AM JOURNAL

Rolled out of bed. Today my outlook, mood, and/or intentions are:

3 Goals to roll with today and the steps to get there:

1.	2.	3.

A. B. C.	A. B. C.	A. B. C.

Plans for fun, chill-time, or adventures today:

3 Things I am grateful for:

PM JOURNAL

Today I made time to:

o Set the mood

o Cook like a grown up

o Eat like a grown up

o Eat a little less of…

o Practice self-care

o Breathe mindfully

o Enjoy the great outdoors

o Move more

o Connect spiritually

o Connect socially

o Embrace my office space

o Recieve touch

o Experience Happiness

o Honor "me time"

o Visualize my future

o Get a good night's sleep

How much of the good stuff did I get today?

Water/hydration _____

Whole Grains _____

Veggies _____

Fruit _____

Healthy Fat _____

Protein _____

Supplements _____

How did I roll today? Thumbs up, down, or somewhere in between?

Mood _____

Energy _____

Digestion _____

Cravings _____

Today, I appreciate myself because:

Today, I added-in or crowded-out:

Choices that did not really serve or support me:

Happy, grateful, or loving thoughts before bed-time:

AM JOURNAL

Rolled out of bed. Today my outlook, mood, and/or intentions are:

3 Goals to roll with today and the steps to get there:

1.	2.	3.

A. B. C.	A. B. C.	A. B. C.

Plans for fun, chill-time, or adventures today:

3 Things I am grateful for:

PM JOURNAL

Today I made time to:

o Set the mood

o Cook like a grown up

o Eat like a grown up

o Eat a little less of...

o Practice self-care

o Breathe mindfully

o Enjoy the great outdoors

o Move more

o Connect spiritually

o Connect socially

o Embrace my office space

o Recieve touch

o Experience Happiness

o Honor "me time"

o Visualize my future

o Get a good night's sleep

How much of the good stuff did I get today?

Water/hydration _____

Whole Grains _____

Veggies _____

Fruit _____

Healthy Fat _____

Protein _____

Supplements _____

How did I roll today? Thumbs up, down, or somewhere in between?

Mood _____

Energy _____

Digestion _____

Cravings _____

Today, I appreciate myself because:

Today, I added-in or crowded-out:

Choices that did not really serve or support me:

Happy, grateful, or loving thoughts before bed-time:

AM JOURNAL

Rolled out of bed. Today my outlook, mood, and/or intentions are:

3 Goals to roll with today and the steps to get there:

1.	2.	3.

A.	A.	A.
B.	B.	B.
C.	C.	C.

Plans for fun, chill-time, or adventures today:

3 Things I am grateful for:

PM JOURNAL

Today I made time to:

- o Set the mood
- o Cook like a grown up
- o Eat like a grown up
- o Eat a little less of…
- o Practice self-care
- o Breathe mindfully

- o Enjoy the great outdoors
- o Move more
- o Connect spiritually
- o Connect socially
- o Embrace my office space

- o Recieve touch
- o Experience Happiness
- o Honor "me time"
- o Visualize my future
- o Get a good night's sleep

How much of the good stuff did I get today?

Water/hydration _____   Healthy Fat _____

Whole Grains _____   Protein _____

Veggies _____   Supplements _____

Fruit _____

How did I roll today? Thumbs up, down, or somewhere in between?

Mood _____   Digestion _____

Energy _____   Cravings _____

Today, I appreciate myself because:

Today, I added-in or crowded-out:

Choices that did not really serve or support me:

Happy, grateful, or loving thoughts before bed-time:

AM JOURNAL

Rolled out of bed. Today my outlook, mood, and/or intentions are:

3 Goals to roll with today and the steps to get there:

1.	2.	3.

A.	A.	A.
B.	B.	B.
C.	C.	C.

Plans for fun, chill-time, or adventures today:

3 Things I am grateful for:

PM JOURNAL

Today I made time to:

- o Set the mood
- o Cook like a grown up
- o Eat like a grown up
- o Eat a little less of…
- o Practice self-care
- o Breathe mindfully

- o Enjoy the great outdoors
- o Move more
- o Connect spiritually
- o Connect socially
- o Embrace my office space

- o Recieve touch
- o Experience Happiness
- o Honor "me time"
- o Visualize my future
- o Get a good night's sleep

How much of the good stuff did I get today?

Water/hydration _____   Healthy Fat _____

Whole Grains _____   Protein _____

Veggies _____   Supplements _____

Fruit _____

How did I roll today? Thumbs up, down, or somewhere in between?

Mood _____   Digestion _____

Energy _____   Cravings _____

Today, I appreciate myself because:

Today, I added-in or crowded-out:

Choices that did not really serve or support me:

Happy, grateful, or loving thoughts before bed-time:

AM JOURNAL

Rolled out of bed. Today my outlook, mood, and/or intentions are:

3 Goals to roll with today and the steps to get there:

| 1. | 2. | 3. |

A.

B.

C.

A.

B.

C.

A.

B.

C.

Plans for fun, chill-time, or adventures today:

3 Things I am grateful for:

PM JOURNAL

Today I made time to:

o Set the mood
o Cook like a grown up
o Eat like a grown up
o Eat a little less of...
o Practice self-care
o Breathe mindfully

o Enjoy the great outdoors
o Move more
o Connect spiritually
o Connect socially
o Embrace my office space

o Recieve touch
o Experience Happiness
o Honor "me time"
o Visualize my future
o Get a good night's sleep

How much of the good stuff did I get today?

Water/hydration _____
Whole Grains _____
Veggies _____
Fruit _____

Healthy Fat _____
Protein _____
Supplements _____

How did I roll today? Thumbs up, down, or somewhere in between?

Mood _____
Energy _____

Digestion _____
Cravings _____

Today, I appreciate myself because:

Today, I added-in or crowded-out:

Choices that did not really serve or support me:

Happy, grateful, or loving thoughts before bed-time:

AM JOURNAL

Rolled out of bed. Today my outlook, mood, and/or intentions are:

3 Goals to roll with today and the steps to get there:

1.	2.	3.

A. B. C.	A. B. C.	A. B. C.

Plans for fun, chill-time, or adventures today:

3 Things I am grateful for:

PM JOURNAL

Today I made time to:

o Set the mood
o Cook like a grown up
o Eat like a grown up
o Eat a little less of…
o Practice self-care
o Breathe mindfully

o Enjoy the great outdoors
o Move more
o Connect spiritually
o Connect socially
o Embrace my office space

o Recieve touch
o Experience Happiness
o Honor "me time"
o Visualize my future
o Get a good night's sleep

How much of the good stuff did I get today?

Water/hydration ———————————
Whole Grains ———————————
Veggies ———————————
Fruit ———————————

Healthy Fat ———————————
Protein ———————————
Supplements ———————————

How did I roll today? Thumbs up, down, or somewhere in between?

Mood ———————————
Energy ———————————

Digestion ———————————
Cravings ———————————

Today, I appreciate myself because:

Today, I added-in or crowded-out:

Choices that did not really serve or support me:

Happy, grateful, or loving thoughts before bed-time:

AM JOURNAL

Rolled out of bed. Today my outlook, mood, and/or intentions are:

3 Goals to roll with today and the steps to get there:

1.	2.	3.

A. B. C.	A. B. C.	A. B. C.

Plans for fun, chill-time, or adventures today:

3 Things I am grateful for:

PM JOURNAL

Today I made time to:

- o Set the mood
- o Cook like a grown up
- o Eat like a grown up
- o Eat a little less of…
- o Practice self-care
- o Breathe mindfully

- o Enjoy the great outdoors
- o Move more
- o Connect spiritually
- o Connect socially
- o Embrace my office space

- o Recieve touch
- o Experience Happiness
- o Honor "me time"
- o Visualize my future
- o Get a good night's sleep

How much of the good stuff did I get today?

Water/hydration ——————————

Whole Grains ——————————

Veggies ——————————

Fruit ——————————

Healthy Fat ——————————

Protein ——————————

Supplements ——————————

How did I roll today? Thumbs up, down, or somewhere in between?

Mood ——————————

Energy ——————————

Digestion ——————————

Cravings ——————————

Today, I appreciate myself because:

Today, I added-in or crowded-out:

Choices that did not really serve or support me:

Happy, grateful, or loving thoughts before bed-time:

WEEKLY AFTER ACTION REPORT

DATES _____

What's new? What's good?

Energy _____

_____

Digestion _____

_____

Cravings _____

_____

Hair & skin _____

_____

Mouth/teeth/tongue _____

_____

Body shape/body image/weight _____

_____

Breathing _____

_____

Moods _____

_____

Relationships _____

_____

Most nourishing food _____

_____

Most filling non-food _____

_____

Someone I especially appreciate _____

_____

Biggest challenge I faced _____

_____

Primary health concern _____

_____

Greatest success _____

_____

Most fun I had _____

_____

Something that became clear this week _____

_____

Other deep thoughts _____

_____

Next week is gonna roll like this.... _____

_____

2 WEEK CHECK IN

Ask someone special in your life to write you a love letter. Have them write it here, or you can paste it here later. Cherish these words, and reference them for a loving reminder when you so desire.

Just Roll With LOVE....

What does YOUR life look like NOW?

1. Place a dot in each category slice to indicate your level of satisfaction within each area. Place a dot at the center of the circle to indicate dissatisfaction, or on the periphery to indicate satisfaction.

2. Connect the dots to see your Circle of Life.

3. Identify imbalances. Determine where to spend more time and energy to create balance.

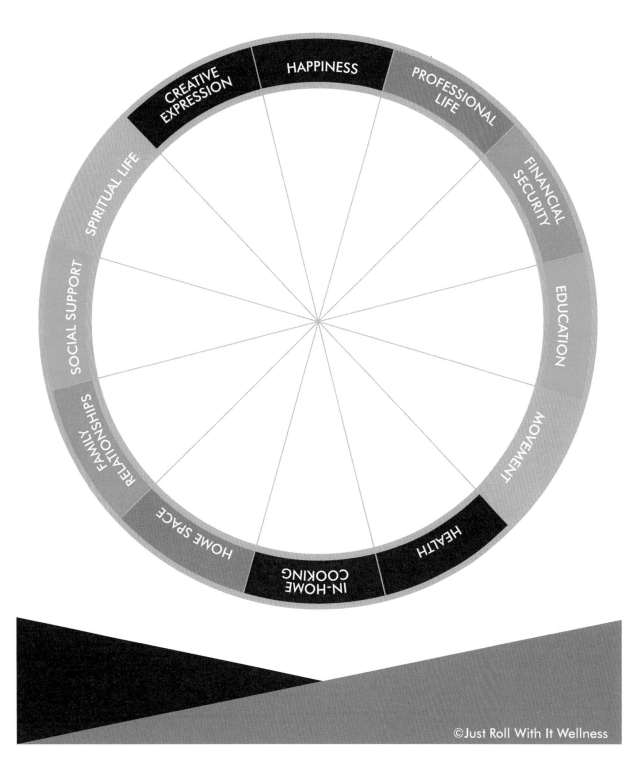

You've come a long way in the last month!

We hope the journey has brought you tremendous joy.

Are you a bit closer to having a strong body, passionate spirit, and a grateful heart?

Then keep rolling with it!

To order another journal, please visit Amazon.com

And remember...

Self-care is not selfish!

Small changes make big differences.

Do your best to flow with your battle rhythms.

Offer yourself both grit and grace.

Reach out to others.

Connect.

Open your mind.

Open your heart.

Be grateful.

Keep going.

Be a light to others.

In gratitude, Sarah & Kate
www.JustRollWithItWellness.com

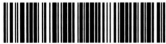

Made in the USA
Lexington, KY
03 February 2018